Awesome, Disgusting Careers

DISGUSTING MEDICAL JOBS

Mary E. Bleck

BLACK RABBIT BOOKS

Hi Jinx is published by Black Rabbit Books
P.O. Box 227, Mankato, Minnesota, 56002.
www.blackrabbitbooks.com

Marysa Storm, editor; Michael Sellner, designer and photo researcher

Names: Bleckwehl, Mary Evanson, author.
Title: Disgusting medical jobs / by Mary E. Bleckwehl.
Description: Mankato, Minnesota : Black Rabbit Books, [2023] | Series: Hi jinx. Awesome, disgusting careers | Includes bibliographical references and index. | Audience: Ages: 8-12 | Audience: Grades: 4-6 | Summary: "Let readers explore the awesome, disgusting medical jobs that keep their world running smoothly through witty, conversational text, fun facts, and critical thinking questions that'll have them laughing and learning"- Provided by publisher.
Identifiers: LCCN 2020030430 (print) | LCCN 2020030431 (ebook) | ISBN 9781623106836 (hardcover) | ISBN 9781644665503 (paperback) | ISBN 9781623106898 (ebook)
Subjects: LCSH: Medical personnel-Juvenile literature. | Medicine-Vocational guidance-Juvenile literature.
Classification: LCC R690 .B596 2022 (print) | LCC R690 (ebook) | DDC 610.73/7069-dc23
LC record available at https://lccn.loc.gov/2020030430
LC ebook record available at https://lccn.loc.gov/2020030431

Image Credits

Alamy: Tim Gainey, 12; iStock: Big_Ryan, Cover; FrankRamspott, Cover, 16; jamesbenet, 8; SDI Productions, 4; simonkr, 10–11; South_agency, Cover, 16; Shutterstock: Aleksei Martynov, 15; Alexander_P, 18–19; Alica in Wonderland, Cover, 8, 21; Arcady, 17; blambca, 15; BluedarkArt, 2–3, 23; chompoo, 15; Christos Georghiou, 21; Gerain0812, 7; Irina Rogova, 16; Jeff Morin, 15; LoopAll, Cover, 1, 5, 6, 20; Lorelyn Medina, 2–3; Memo Angeles, 9, 13, 15, 19, 20; Naeblys, 12; Pasko Maksim, 6, 23, 24; picoStudio, 4, 10; Pitju, 21; Pushkin, 15; Ron Dale, 5, 6, 20; Rvector, 19; Sakan.p, 8; Teeradej, 16; thirawatana phaisalratana, 8; totallypic, 12; ymphotos, 7

CONTENTS

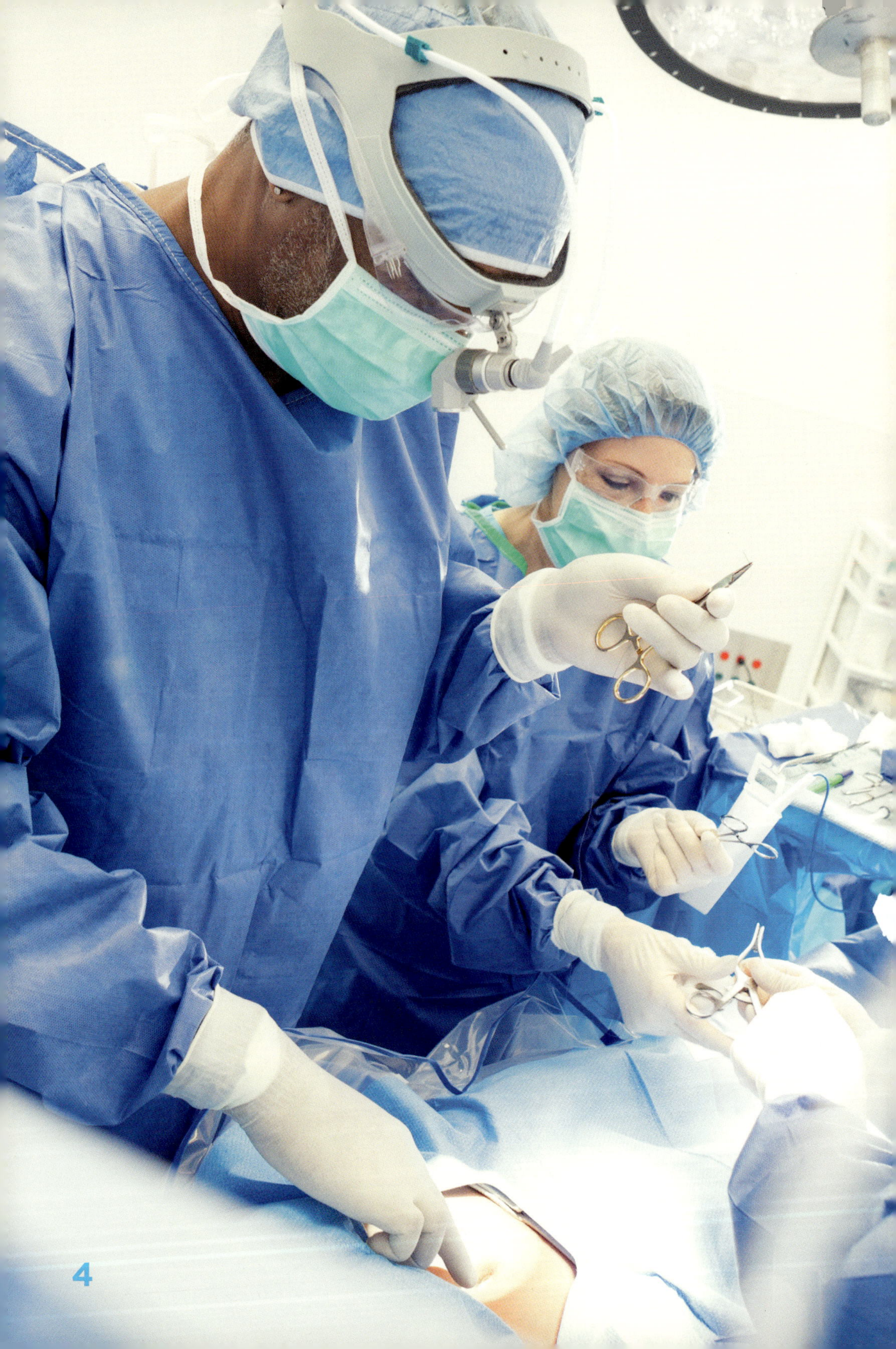

Chapter 1
BODY WORK

Medical workers keep people safe. They help patients feel better. Most make good money too. But there is some serious yuck involved! We're talking oozing wounds and plenty of blood. Does reading that make you wanna puke? Better grab a bucket before you turn the page!

Chapter 2

THE JOBS

Cosmetic Surgeon

Want a smaller nose? It's a cosmetic surgeon who'll give you one. These doctors change the shapes or sizes of body parts. They suck fat from bellies. They remove sagging skin. Sometimes they **transplant** hair. These jobs are disgusting. But the results can be amazing!

Some doctors freeze away a person's fat.

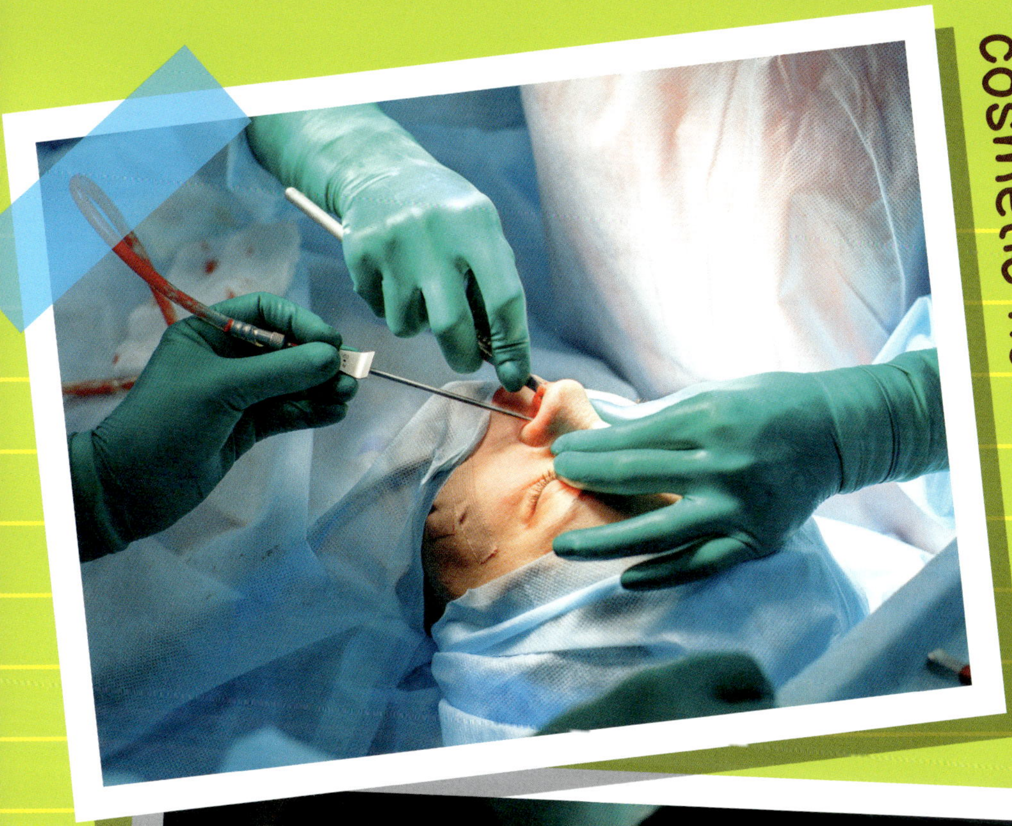

cosmetic nose surgery

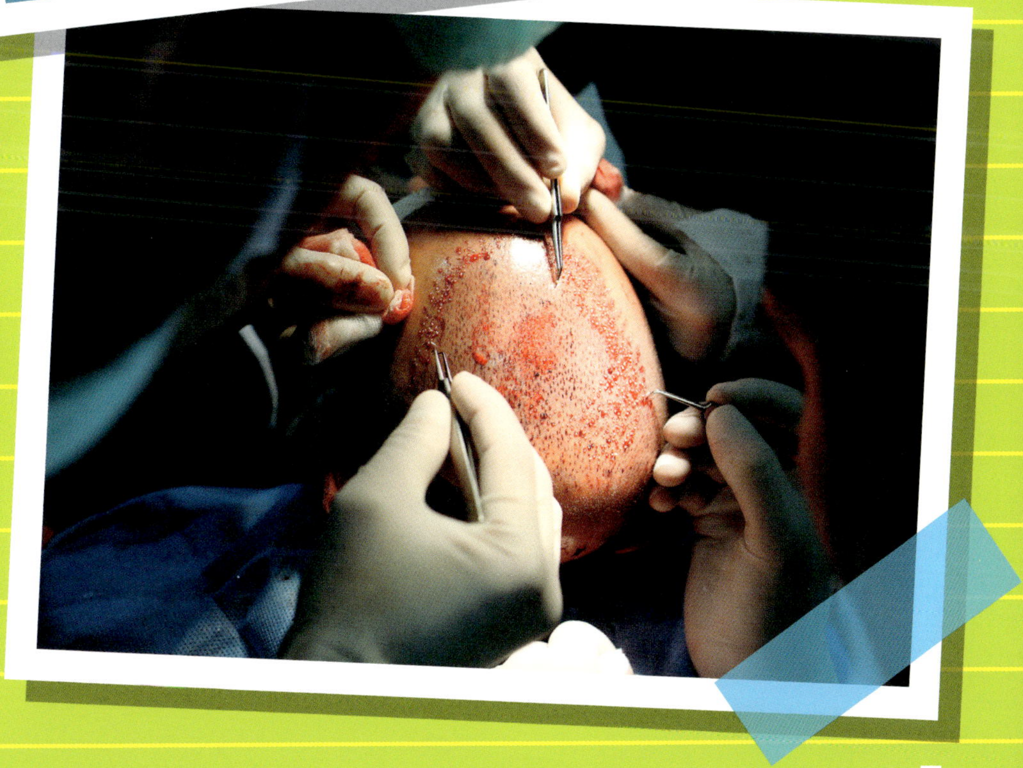

hair transplant

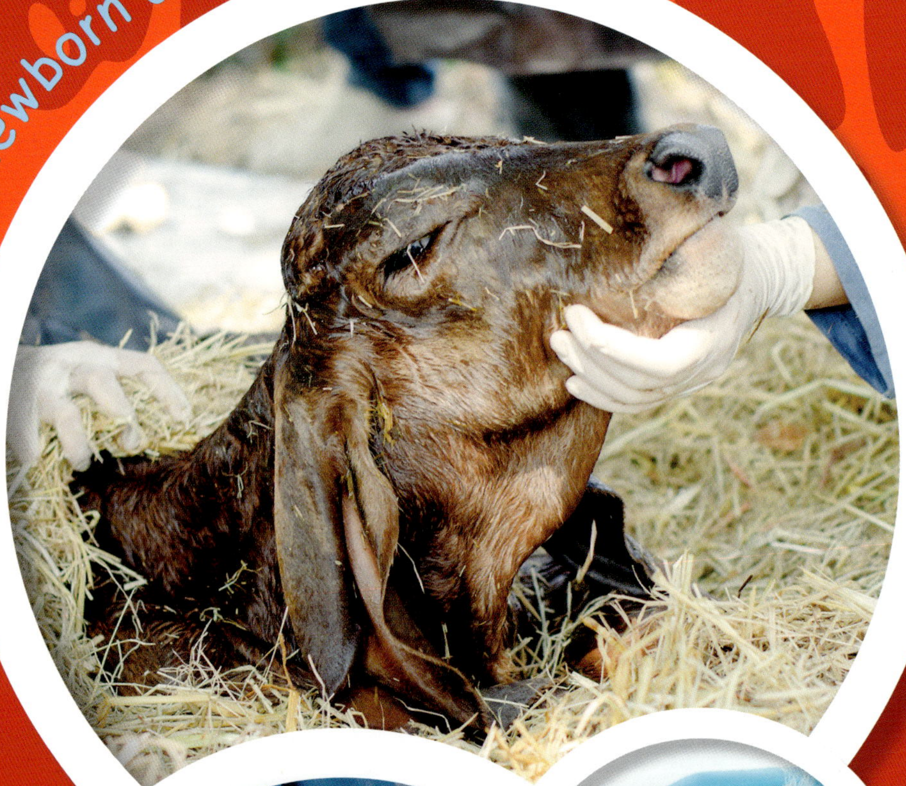

newborn calf

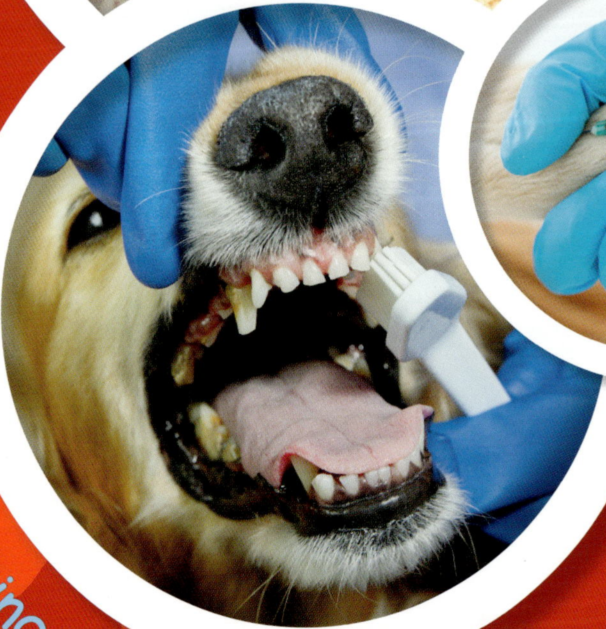

brushing teeth

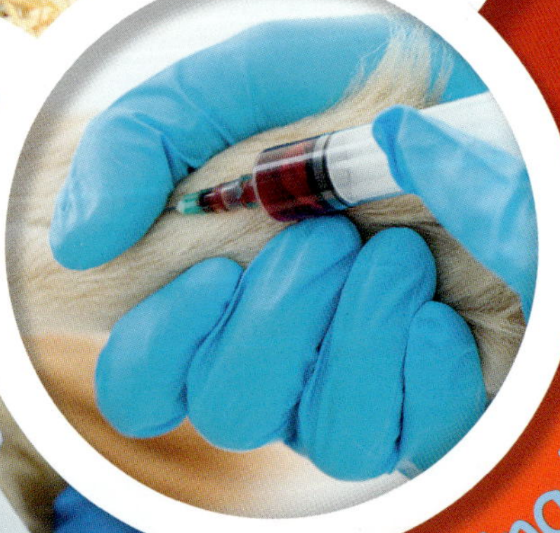

drawing blood

Veterinarian

Vets are animal doctors. And working with animals isn't always cute. Sometimes vets help cows give birth. Other times they **draw** blood or clean animals' teeth. They also deal with pet puke, pee, and poop. These doctors don't reek. But their jobs do.

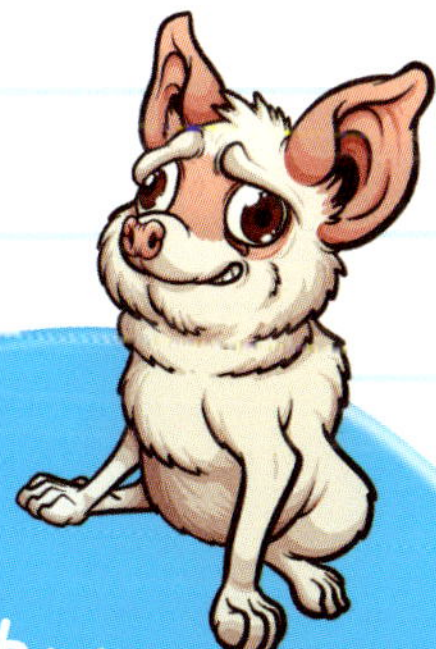

Got a butt-dragging pooch? Its anal glands might be clogged. A vet must drain them.

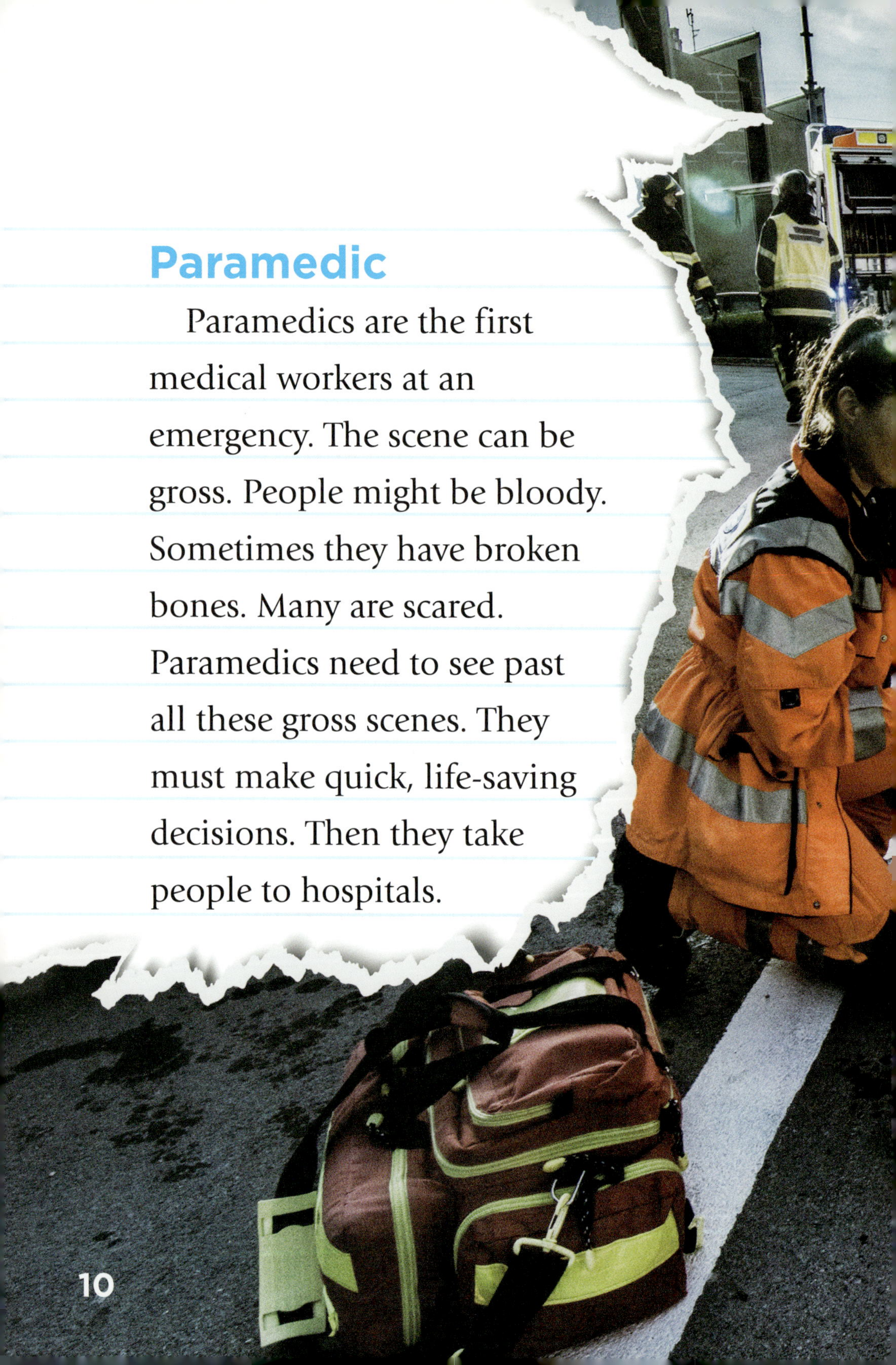

Paramedic

Paramedics are the first medical workers at an emergency. The scene can be gross. People might be bloody. Sometimes they have broken bones. Many are scared. Paramedics need to see past all these gross scenes. They must make quick, life-saving decisions. Then they take people to hospitals.

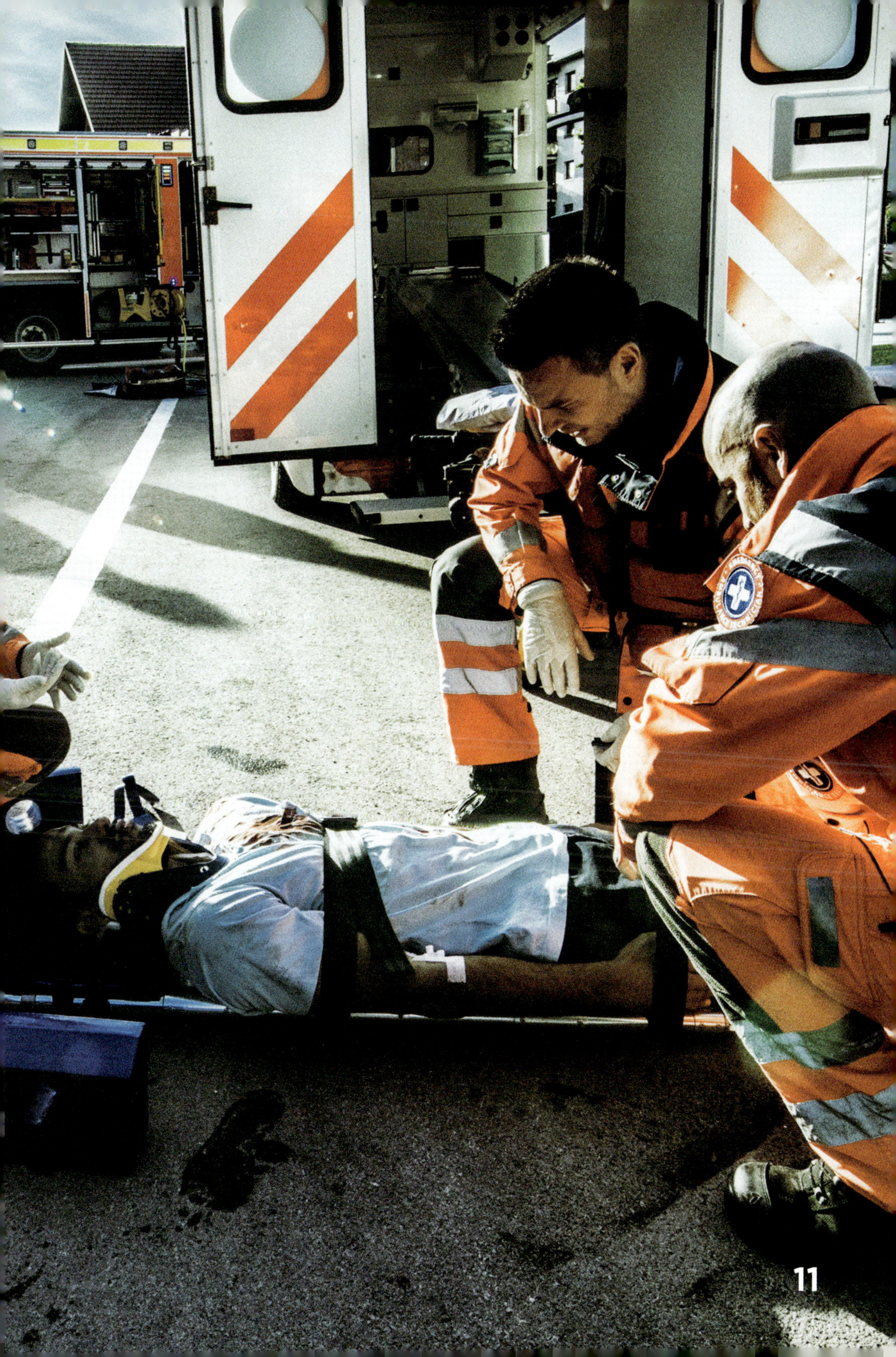

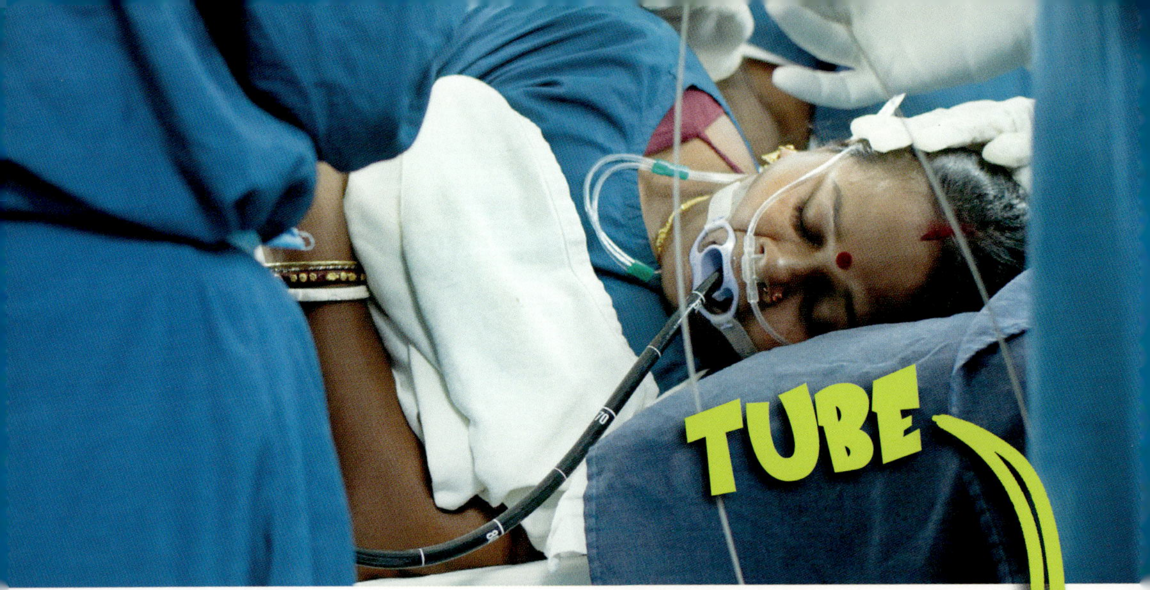
TUBE

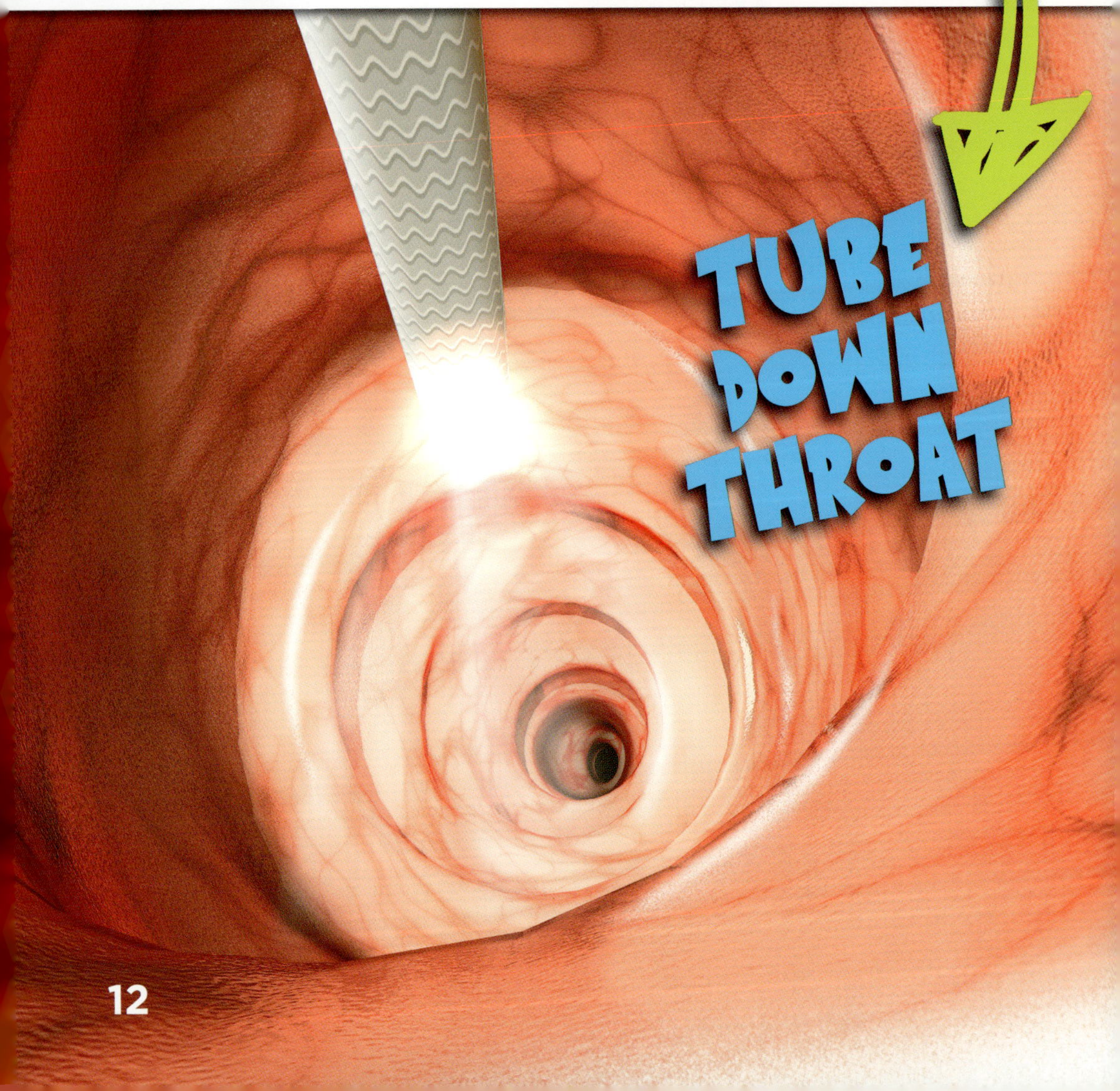
TUBE
DOWN
THROAT

Gastroenterologist

Gastroenterologists are a type of doctor. They focus on **digestive** health. That means they deal with some of our embarrassing parts. Sometimes they push a tube up someone's bottom. They do this to check out the **intestinal** track. Other times they send tubes down throats to see if there's a problem. Stinky smells and bare butts are all part of this work.

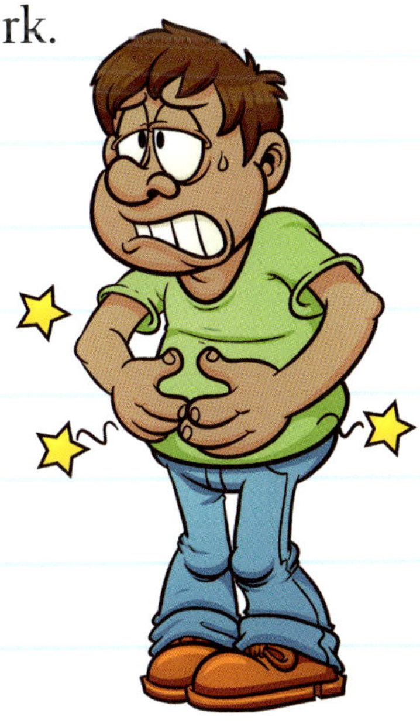

Fart Sniffer

Stench alert! Some people work as professional smellers. These workers spot diseases by taking a whiff of our natural gas. Yes, we're talking about sniffin' farts. Does your fart smell fishy or meaty? There might be a **tumor**. Some farts are over-the-top stinky. Those mean something could be wrong with a person's guts.

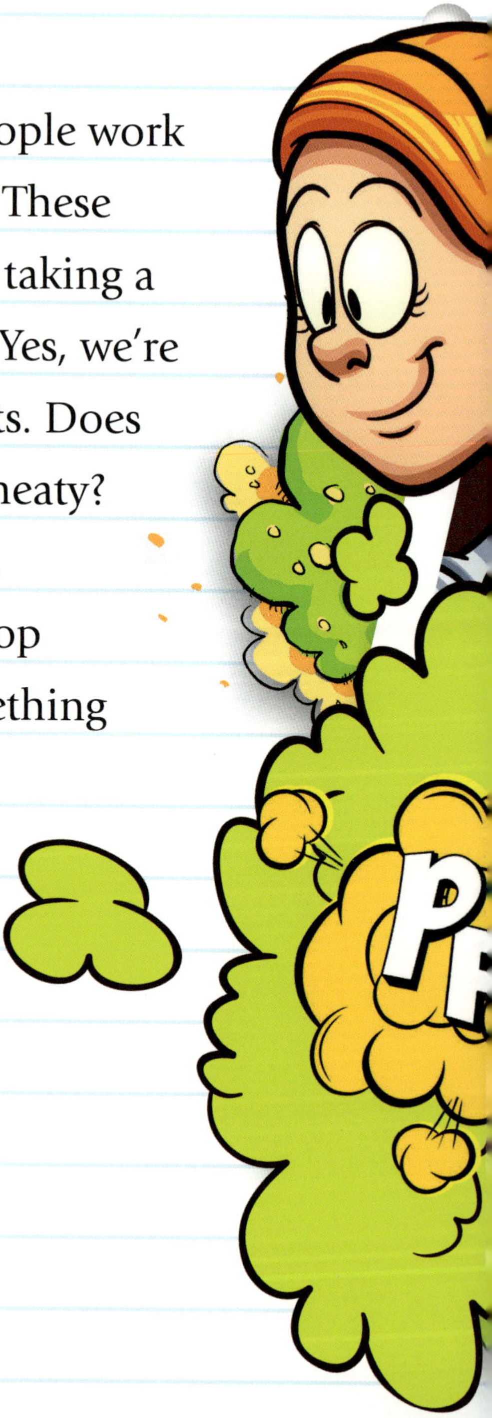

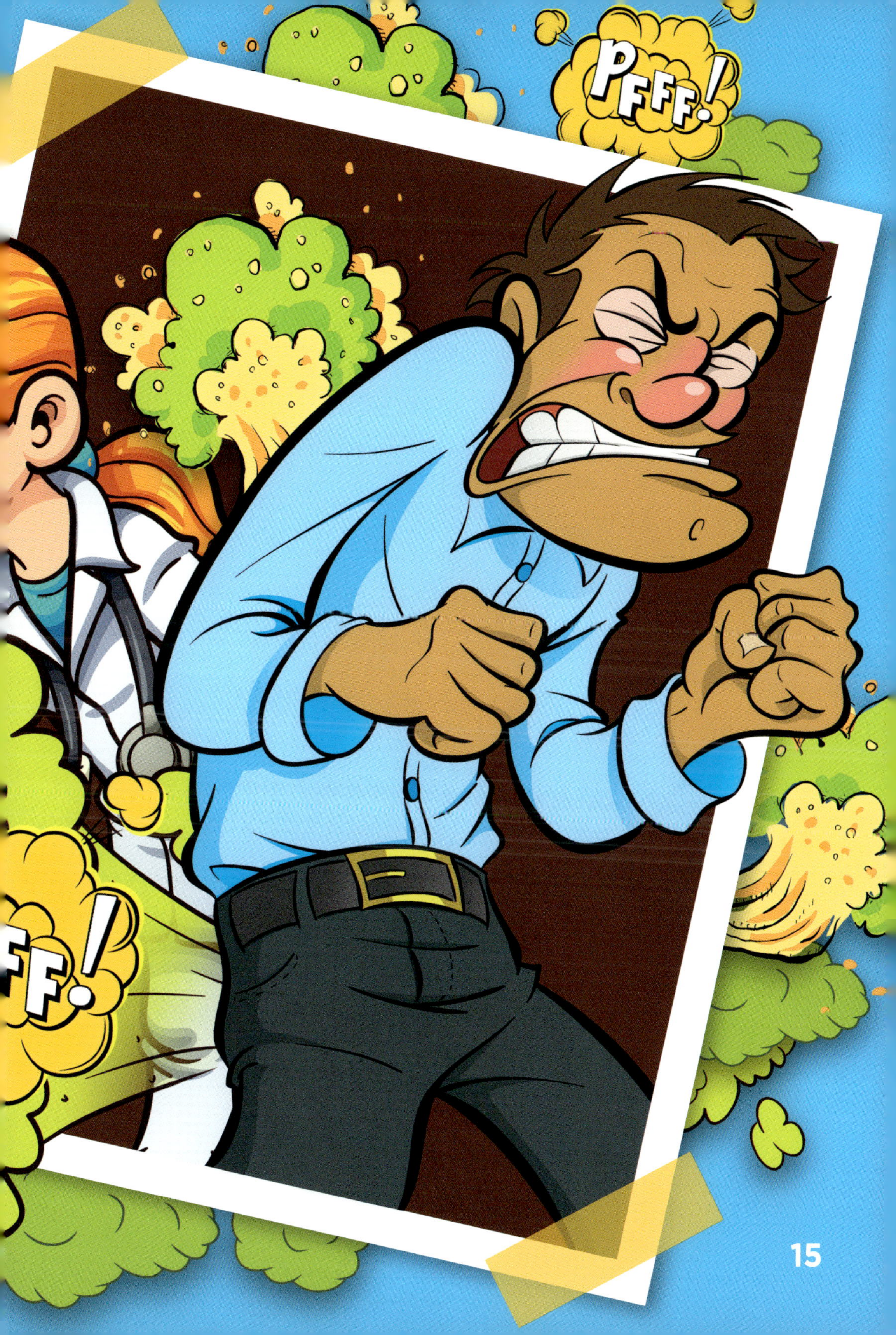
PFFF!
FF!

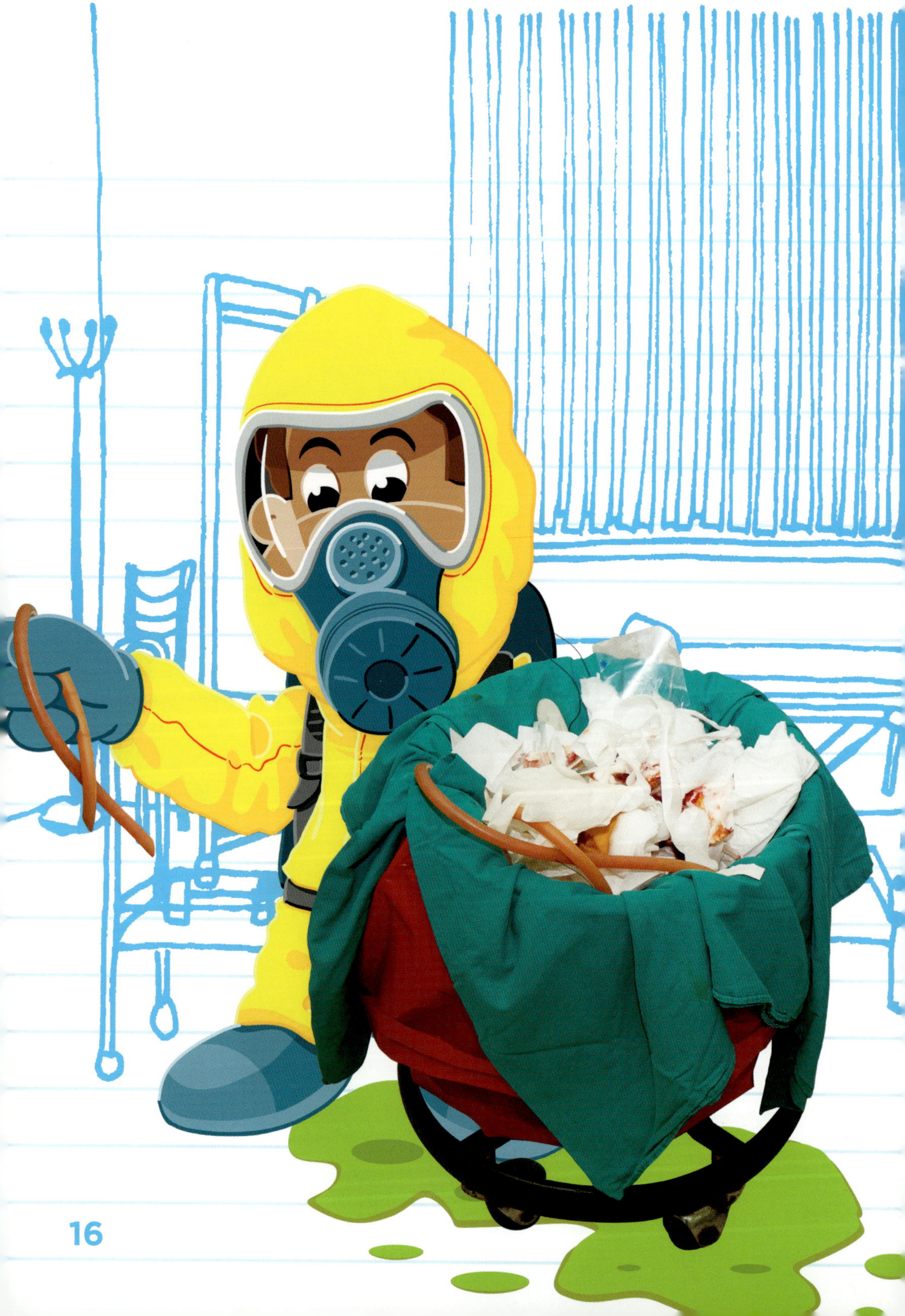

Medical Waste Disposal Worker

Medical waste disposal workers take care of the waste created by hospitals. That includes body parts! Often, they burn this waste. They throw other waste, such as needles, away. It's gross. But someone has to do it.

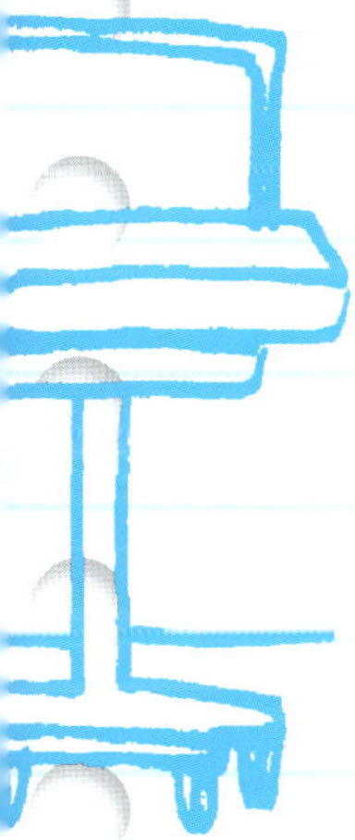

In 2015, a Florida hospital made a mistake. It threw a leg away. The leg ended up in a landfill.

Medical Examiner

Yuck! Medical examiners are doctors who perform autopsies. An autopsy is cutting into a person's body to understand why they died. These doctors dig through fat and organs. They might need to fish bullets from someone's brain. These doctors must think like detectives.

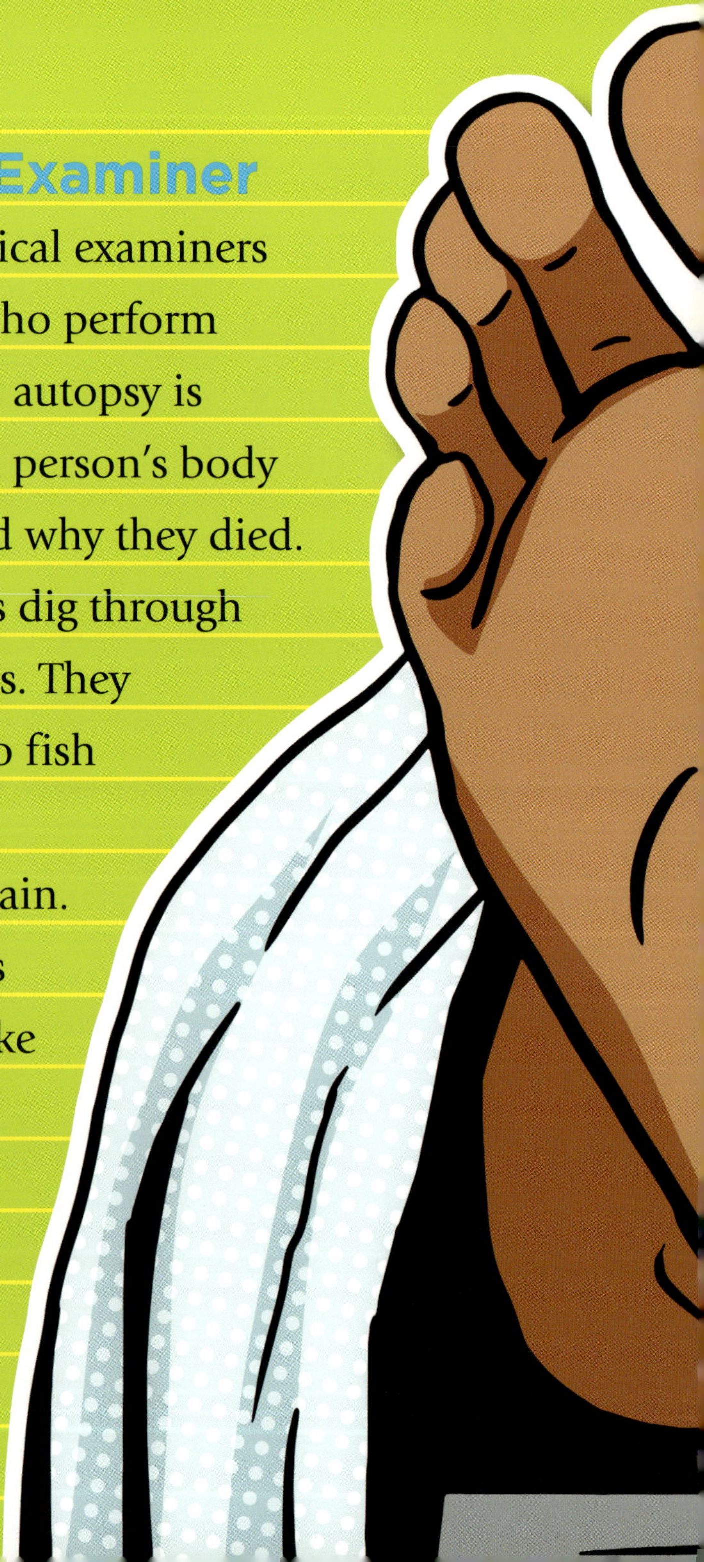

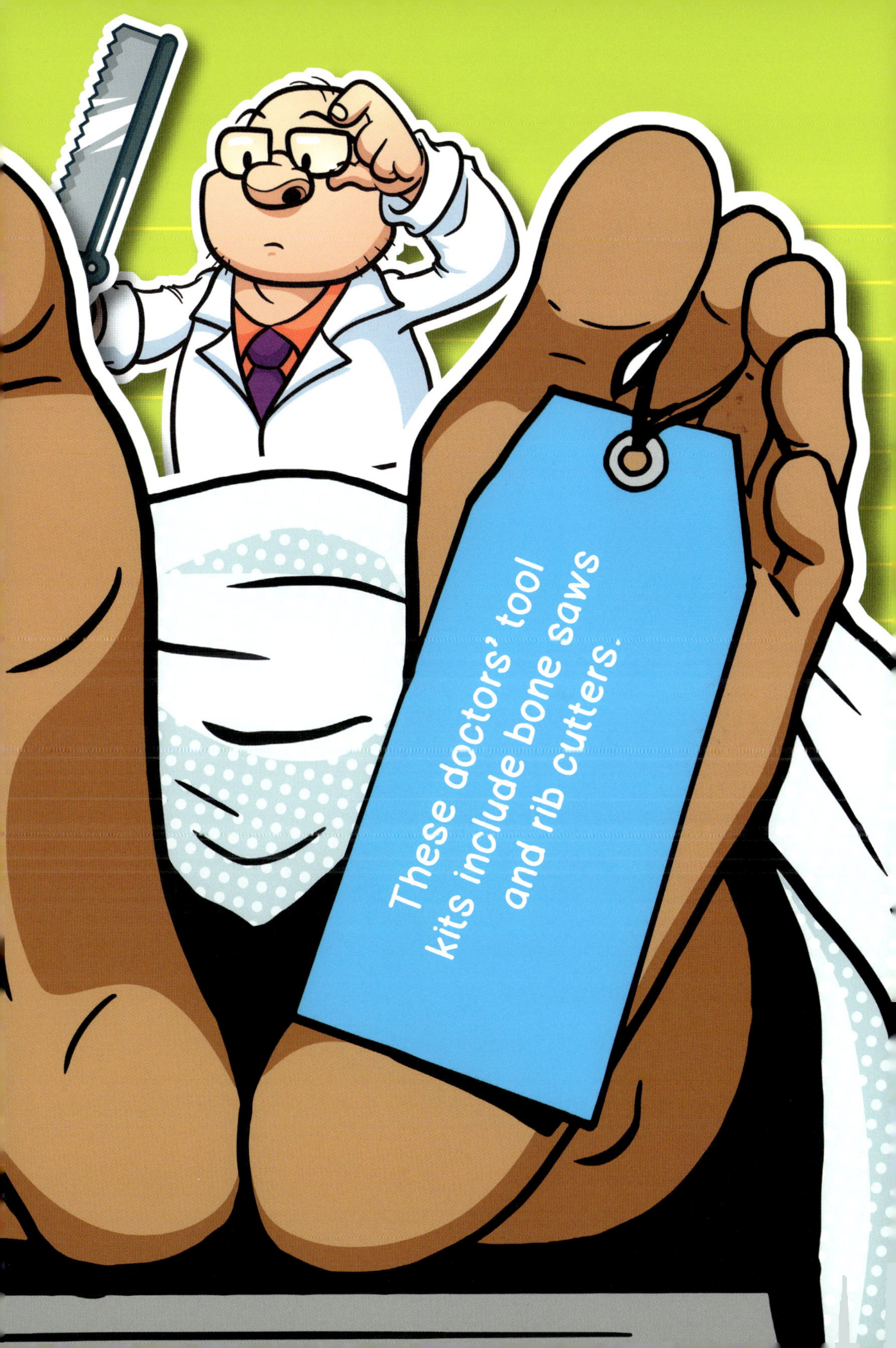
These doctors' tool kits include bone saws and rib cutters.

Chapter 3
GET IN ON THE HI JINX

Most medical jobs require a lot of training. Doctors need medical **degrees** and years of specialized training. Paramedics need at least a two-year degree. Other workers are trained on the job. As for fart sniffers, having a good sense of smell is just one requirement. Which job do you want?

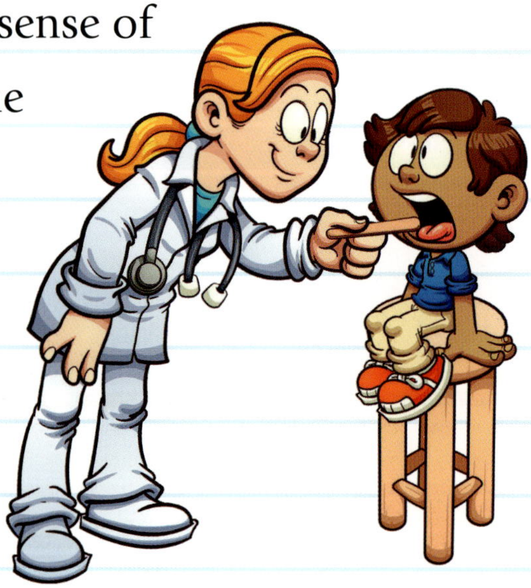

Take It One Step More

1. Would you rather be a doctor that takes care of people or animals? Why?
2. What would be the most interesting thing about being a medical examiner?
3. Which job in this book do you think is the grossest? Why?

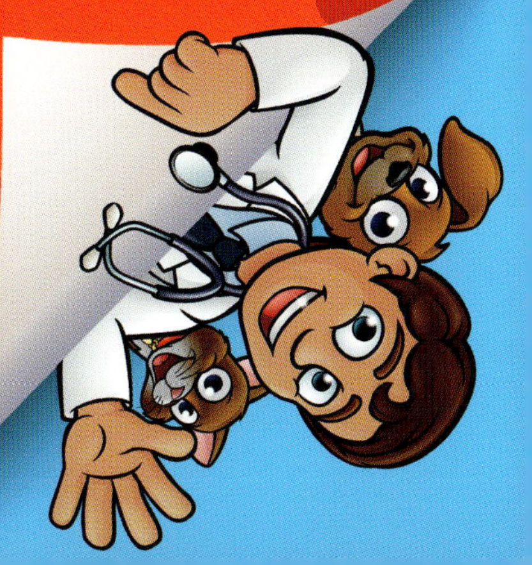

GLOSSARY

anal (EYN-l)—relating to or involving the lower opening of the digestive tract

degree (dih-GREE)—a title given by a college or university

digestive (dy-JEST-iv)—having the power to cause or help digestion

draw (DRAW)—to bring or pull out

intestinal (in-TES-tuh-nl)—relating to or part of the digestive system where most food is digested

transplant (trans-PLANT)—to move an organ or tissue from one part or individual to another

tumor (TOO-muhr)—an abnormal growth of tissue

LEARN MORE

BOOKS

Learmonth, Amanda, and Elise Gaignet. *I Like Helping People ... What Jobs Are There?* That's a Job? Tulsa, OK: Kane Miller, a Division of EDC Publishing, 2021.

Mattern, Joanne. *Disgusting Jobs.* That's Disgusting! Minneapolis: Kaleidoscope, 2020.

Nickel, Scott. *World's Grossest Jobs.* Minneapolis: Lerner Publications, 2021.

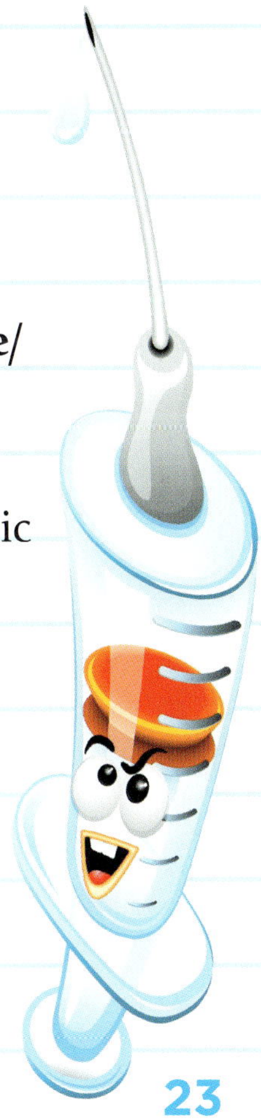

WEBSITES

15 Facts about the Human Body!
www.natgeokids.com/nz/discover/science/general-science/15-facts-about-the-human-body/

Emergency Medical Technicians & Paramedic
www.sciencebuddies.org/science-engineering-careers/health/emergency-medical-technicians-paramedic

Medical Doctor Facts for Kids
kids.kiddle.co/Medical_doctor

INDEX